Also by Dr. Stenbeck

Available from the usual on-line source

Books
Healing Yourself -- The Holistic Approach
  [An introduction to Holistic Self-healing.]

Heal Yourself Right Now!
  [The Seven Priority Organ Levels for
  effective Nutritional/Holistic Treatment of
  all organs.]

The 22 Unique Body Types
  (for Health and Weight Loss)

Q & A to Identify Your Body Type (Booklet)
  [Individual Type booklets are also available

Booklets
(Step-by-step instructions on healing yourself)

  #1 Start Healing with Positive Thinking
  #2 Mastering Positive Feelings for Health!
  #3 Spiritual Balance and Your Healing

The Exesthesic Body Type

Representing one of the 22 Body Types first described by Victor Rocine around 1900

The Cher, Sarah Jessica Parker Celebrity Body Type

For Kaye,
there at the beginning with Doc Severn,
and for Liberty,
continuing the holistic healing journey…

Disclaimer

The information in this book is for educational purposes only and is not a substitute for medication, diets, or other medical care. The diets do not treat diseases or medical conditions, and are an adjunct to your orthodox health care.

The author and publisher accept no responsibility for any misuse of the information within. If you have any physical problem, food allergy, emotional disorder, or disease, common sense dictates that you consult with a physician before changing your diet, taking nutritional supplements, or following the advice given here.

———

About the Author

Educated in New Zealand and in the U.S.A., Dr. Stenbeck attained B.Sc. (NZ), M.S., and D.C. degrees. His holistic healing methods have been profiled in magazines (Esquire, McLean's, Playgirl, the Atlanta Constitution), and on TV in the USA and in Canada. He was the main contributor to the Warner Book, _The Eye/Body Connection_ by Jessica Maxwell that focused on the holistic healing relationships between the iris structure and organ genetics.

In the 1970-80's he was elected Fellow, Royal Society of Health, London; Fellow, American Association of Chemists; Member, American Association of Clinical Chemists; and Affiliate, Royal Society of Medicine, London. He studied naturopathy and Body Types with Dr. Bernard Jensen and Dr. Clifford Severn, and has practiced in medical partnerships where patients received the joint benefits of medical and holistic healing.

He is a member of Self-Realization Fellowship. To receive advice on any health issue from a holistic viewpoint, or to receive help with your body type, see his web site: *DrStenbeck.net*

Contents

* * *

The Exesthesic Body Type and Food Guide   1

* * *

The 22 Body Types:
Celebrity Examples

This Booklet contains the **Exesthesic** type.
See <u>The 22 Unique Body Types</u> for all type
descriptions.]

Thin Types

Atrophic
: Woody Allen / Audrey Hepburn
Stan Laurel / Calista Flockheart

Exesthesic
: Cher / Sarah Jessica Parker
(Female type only)

Marasmic
: President Obama / Princess Diana
James Stewart / Kate Blanchard

Neurogenic
: J.K. Simmons / Joan Rivers
Jon Cryer / Marin Hinle

Pathoferic
: (No celebrity males)
Blythe Danner / Gwyneth Paltrow

Sillevitic
: David Bowie / Shirley MacLaine
Rod Stewart / Carol Channing

Muscle Types

Calciferic   *Michael Jordan / Angelica Huston*
Abraham Lincoln / Robin Wright

Carbogenic   *George Clooney / Lady Gaga*
Pres. G. Bush, Jr. / Meg Ryan

Desmogenic   *Marlon Brando / Loni Anderson*
Daniel Craig / Tina Turner

Eldic   *Ross Perot / Hillary Clinton*
Peter Falk / Sigourney Weaver

Myogenic   *Pres. Bill Clinton / Sharon Stone*
Pres. John Kennedy / Julia Roberts

Nervimotive   *Frank Sinatra / Elizabeth Taylor*
Mark Wahlberg / Natalie Wood

Nitropheric   *Ben Affleck / Ava Gardner*
Kirk Douglas / Kate Winslet

Pallinomic   *Pres. Donald Trump /*
Attorney General Janet Reno
Bill O'Reilly (Fox) / Jane Russell

Fat Types

Barotic	*Robin Williams / 'Mrs.Doubtfire'* *Elton John / William Conrad*
Carboferic	*Bill Murray / Roseanne* *Billy Gardell / Melissa McCarthy*
Hydripheric	*John Goodman / Shelly Winters* *Wayne Knight / Jennifer Holliday*
Isogenic	*Einstein / Oprah Winfrey* *Phillip S .Hoffman / Queen Victoria*
Lipopheric	*Rush Limbaugh / Rosie O'Donnell* *Chris Christie / Camryn Manheim*
Oxypheric	*Winston Churchill / Orsen Welles* *Ella Fitzgerald / Gerry Spence*
Pargenic	*Burt Reynolds / Katey Segal* *Ron Perlman / Kirstey Alley*

Succinct Quote on Human Types

From Victor Rocine, who first described discrete body types around 1900.

"A type is an order of people that differentiates and distinguishes itself by a general and similar form, brain-formation, chemistry, structure, build, immunity, tendencies, predisposition, resemblance, skin-pigment, and type characteristics based on observation and analogy.

"Or, in other words, people of a given type are similar physically and like-minded as if they were brothers and sisters—that is what type means.

"Everything in nature is made according to plan. Man only discovers that plan and gives it a name. The zoologist has not made the animals—he has only described the plan adopted by the wonderful Creator, and named the classes, sub-classes, etc.

"How important type research will be to humanity, time alone will make known."

———

Prologue

The esteemed scientist J. J. Berzelius, discoverer of several chemical elements, inspired Victor Rocine to research body types and to investigate the correlation between types and their diseases. Around 1890-1910, Rocine privately published his original findings on the mineral basis of different body types, and this present book exists because of his brilliant insights.

For many years, I studied with Dr. Clifford Severn who had been a personal student of Victor Rocine on body types, naturopathy, herbology, iris analysis, diet, and nutritional healing methods. He had a successful career as a lecturer and healer, and was one of those rare athletes with complete muscle control over his body. I saw him under a spotlight at 85 years of age, contracting and rippling every individual muscle in his perfectly developed body. Field-Marshal Jan Smuts, the WWII South African Prime Minister, devoted a full chapter of his autobiography to how Severn's healing methods had saved his life. In the 1950's, *Life* magazine did a four-page spread on Severn and his family. Fame he had.

Another Rocine student I studied with, Dr. Bernard Jensen wrote of Rocine's body type research and nutritional methods in his privately published book *The Chemistry of Man*.

This book is deeply rooted in Rocine's original work, and with that of Herbert Shelton, M.D., Ph.D. (at Harvard University in the 1930's). I integrated their research with newer dietary and nervous system data along with celebrity examples of each type, hopefully, making this material easier to digest and more entertaining for the reader.

Gayelord Hauser, another Rocine student I knew, was a celebrated health book author. He wrote a popular book on Rocine's types in the 1940's, *Types and Temperaments;* reputedly, he also introduced yogurt to the western world.

This book exists because of Rocine's creative brilliance and original discoveries in natural healing.

▶ *Rocine: "The soul creates the body type."*

Rocine taught that the soul chooses a body type and brain to live in, thus presenting different experiences and life lessons to master. Why were *you* born the way you are?

That is something to think about, especially if it is true! What would your soul purpose be to live in a particular body type. I provide some thoughts on this issue in each type description and try to assess from my experience with your type the particular lessons of life presented therein.

Rocine was as brilliant in his way as an Abraham Lincoln, Michael Jordan, Michael Phelps, Tony Robbins, or a Daniel Day Lewis—all *calciferic* types—rare, leaders, innovative, brilliant, and highly intelligent in their different fields of endeavor.

Celebrity examples exist for most types, not a duplicate of you, but someone who has your essence in their body-mind individuality. Knowing your type allows you to become a better you!

The celebrity examples provide further help in identifying your body type.

▶ *Rocine's classic findings are the backbone of this book. Integrated with Sheldon's research and with other dietary and food issues including mental, emotional, and spiritual attributes,*

Many people take nutritional supplements and try different diets without a doctor's advice. If this is your choice, use common sense, listen to body responses, and discontinue any allergic reactions to foods or nutritional substances.

———

The Exesthesic Body Type

* * *

"You may also have a physical or psychological feature not representative of your type such as height, weight, appearance, talent, weakness, strength, etc., due to biochemical errors, environmental influences, racial or cultural differences, and congenital or genetic issues. Nevertheless, the type identification of the average person is usually clear."

— *Victor Rocine*

Exesthesic Type Celebrity Examples

If you think this is your type, be sure to look at **on-line photographs** *of these examples. Look for general similarities to yourself. Note that sub-types cause the differences in appearance between members of the same type. You are a female-only and a rare body type.*

ACTING

[There are few examples.]

Cher
Sarah Jessica Parker *("Sex and the City")*
Teri Garr *("Close Encounters of the Third Kind")*
("Friends)

You already know something about this type from their public persona and appearance, whether from seeing them yourself or from the celebrity examples. Blend such insights with the type descriptions and the types of your family and friends to discern their presence in your midst!

It is noteworthy that I have met only a few females of this type in my whole life. I knew one male *exesthesic* who eventually had a transgender operation.

Read the types, and if still confused, see *Appendix A,* for the personal type identification request from my website: *DrStenbeck.net*

———

Exesthesic Type Questionnaire

These questions describe the generic type, and not specifically you! If any question ever applied to you, then choose the True answer!

For Question 1 only:

A = True	*B = Maybe*	*C = Untrue*
15 points	*7 points*	*1 point*

1. Physically identify with celebrity example____

Then

A = True	*B = Maybe*	*C = Untrue*
5 points	*3 points*	*1 point*

---

2. Height is usually close to: 5'6-5'11   ____
3. Usual weight close to 125-165 pounds ____
4. Shapely, slender or medium-sized body ____
5. Honest, ethical, and practical   ____
6. Oval face usually (hairline to chin)   ____
7. Hair is healthy and/or beautiful with natural brown or chestnut colors   ____
8. More likely to be school cheer-leaders than athletes   ____
9. Attractive, delicate, lovely skin; may not perspire; tend to flush easily   ____
10. Often considered beautiful, graceful; attractive figures, long legs   ____

11. Teeth are white, medium-sized, small,
    narrow, and closely packed   _____
12. Strong sensual nature: attract men
    like bees to honey   _____
13. Good management ability   _____
14. Desire cooked sulfur foods: cabbage,
    cauliflower, garlic, broccoli, etc.   _____
15. Moderate sexual drive (desire quality
    not quantity)   _____
16. Have angry episodes   _____
17. Have high self: confidence and image   _____
18. Enjoy socializing and conversing   _____
19. Periodic aches, pains, or numbness
    in the stomach, chest, joints, or eyes   _____
20. Intelligent, talented, creative   _____
21. Eyes attractive, bright, large, blue,
    hazel, or brown   _____
22. Have a medium to large bust   _____
23. Normal sized chin with sloping jaws   _____
24. Difficulty with arduous studies   _____
25. Ethical, sincere, and exclusive nature   _____
26. Mouth often smaller than average,
    never large (upper lip thinner, drawn)   _____
27. Muscles are moderately strong   _____
28 Long, slender, and graceful extremities   _____
29. Long, lean back; sloping shoulders   _____
30. May have heavy hips; weight easily
    controlled; high waistline   _____
31. Spine, tendons, joints easily stressed   _____
32. Trustworthy, responsible   _____
33. Eyelids vulnerable to infections   _____
34. Industrious and hard working   _____

35. Have artistic skills (not scientists)   _____
36. Very assertive, may upset others   _____
37. Have domestic skills: home-making, sewing, etc.   _____
38. Inclined to be optimistic, assertive, and never passive   _____
39. Distinctive soprano voice   _____
40. Responsible, efficient, and practical   _____
41. Strong commitment to loved ones, friends, or business partners'   _____
42. Vulnerable to getting upset or angry   _____
43. Have a strong sense of being cautious   _____
44. Highly developed sense of family   _____
45. Mind is very active; strong opinions   _____
46. Tend to be unforgiving if offended   _____
47. Nervousness is very common   _____
48. Tend to seek and need sympathy   _____
49. Aches and pains left side of body   _____
50. Dislike loud noises, electrical storms, heated rooms, cold, and heavy work   _____
51. Rarely inclined to science, medicine, or the professions   _____
52. Small circle of friends (are cautious)   _____
53. Crave love and affection (co-dependent tendency)   _____
54. Rarely athletic   _____

▶ *The type questionnaire pinpoints the major features of that type: if the celebrity examples are unhelpful, you may be an unusual variant (in which case ignore the celebrity issue and give yourself 7 points on Question 1).*

Scoring

For question #1:

A response: give 15 points = _____
B response: give 7 points = _____
C response: give 1 points = _____

For questions #2—54:

A response: give 5 points = _____
B response: give 3 points = _____
C response: give 1 point = _____
Total of the above points = _____

Interpretation

135—265: PROBABLY Exesthesic type
70—134: POSSIBLY Exesthesic type
<70: NOT Exesthesic type

The Exesthesic Type

Rocine: "Exesthesic means, 'the throwing out of feelings'." You utilize more food sulfur than any other type making you volatile, expressive, and nervous. You are a mental type. A female-only type.

———

In a manner similar to the *nervimotive* type you express your feelings as felt. Eating *cooked* sulfur foods like cabbage, cauliflower, onions, garlic, broccoli, turnips, and Brussels sprouts undermines your health.

You may have strong masculine skills and when necessary are able to be tough, dynamic, commanding, authoritative, action-oriented, and to take control of your life. You are of medium-height or tall (never short), and proportionally built. You have a highly developed and difficult to conceal sensuality that attracts men like bees to honey. This is one of your life challenges: to understand how your sensuality and beauty magnetizes males— noticed later is your excellent brain! You are poised and graceful.

▶ *Rocine: "Sulfur is the agent of soul expression…no sulfur, no sensation, no soul communication with the body, no sense, no life, no soul expression. You need raw sulfur foods."*

––––––

Physical Similarity to Other Types

The *myogenic* person (Michelle Pfeiffer) is of medium-height or tall, lean, lovely, stronger, and outgoing.

The *pathoferic* woman (Gwyneth Paltrow) may be pretty or lovely, with a slim build, more introverted, with hidden deep feelings.

The *sillevitic* woman (Florence Henderson) may also be pretty or lovely, with brown or fair hair, and is very outgoing, happy, smiling, and optimistic.

––––––

Average Height and Weight

5'6-5'11   125-165 pounds (female only)

––––––

Exesthesic Type Description

The type description represents how you appear in everyday society. You may have a sub-type that alters parts of this description. Think of Cher and you will know this type.

Like most thin types, you look younger than your age. Hallmarks of your type are grace, femininity, intelligence, talent, sensuality, creativity, and verbal expression. You have long legs and a lovely figure, but aging may provide an extra 10-30 pounds of fat.

Head — You usually have an oval face, and an oval head from front to back when viewed on profile, Cher being a classic example. (Some *marasmic* women also have this feature).

Hair — You usually have beautiful, luxuriant, black, or brown hair.

Eyes — Your eyes are attractive, large, and brown or blue; the eyelids may suffer with minor infections and sties.

▶ *You may have many symptoms (see later list) due to toxic elimination from excessive eating of cooked sulfur foods.*

Ears — The ears are of medium-size and shape.

Nose — Your nose is small to medium-sized.

Face — You have a lovely and delicate face, long and oval from the hairline to the chin with subtle cheek bones. A normal chin with sloping jaws is characteristic.

Mouth, Lips, and Voice — Normal-sized lips are usual although the upper lip may become thinner and drawn with age. You have a high pitched, unique, and distinctive soprano voice.

Teeth — Your teeth are usually strong, small, narrower than average, and aligned closely together.

Skin — Your skin is delicate, sensitive, and may be beautiful. A normal tissue sulfur level gives you healthy skin without body odor. You may smell of sulfur (from cooked sulfur food intake).

Neck — A long and graceful neck is usual.

Chest — The bust is usually medium-sized or large.

Back and Shoulders — A long thin back with gentle sloping shoulders is usual.

Hips and Abdomen — You may carry a few extra pounds on the hips. Your waistline is high on the body.

Arms and Legs — Long, slender, graceful, strong extremities are typical.

Joints — Your ligaments, tendons, joints, and back are vulnerable to damage: scoliosis may occur.

————

Exesthesic Personality Traits

If you are this type many, but not all, of the following characteristics are present—you may have overcome or moderated the negatives, but recognize that you once had several of them.

Positive Qualities

You may have many of the following traits:

- Have great charm
- Intelligent, graceful
- High self-confidence
- Honest verbal expression

- Reasonable and usually helpful
- Friendly, lively, polite, flirtatious
- Honest, sincere, cautious, responsible
- Active mind, studious, excellent memory
- Assertive, high family love and commitments
- Refined, cultured, graceful, noble, ethical, honest, aristocratic
- Sensual (but not overtly sexual), love is periodic: it comes and goes

Potential Challenges

You may have evolved from, or not experienced, these general faults so do not dwell on them.

▶ *Rocine: "You blow off your feelings verbally. When unhealthy you have a tendency to hysteria or to having 'volcanic' emotional eruptions."*

- Proud, jealous, extravagant, moody, changeable
- Easily irritated, well-meaning, but moody, emotional
- May have 'mental storms' (from excess sulfur intake)
- Odd pains or numbness in the stomach or other organs

- You appear nervous, and tend to seek sympathy from others
- You may suffer from peculiar complaints related to excess cooked sulfur food intake
- Dislike of loud noises, electrical storms, heated rooms, cold moisture, and heavy physical work

▶ *If you relate to any of the above challenges doing something to overcome them serves your evolution.*

———

Exesthesic Stress Management

You have weak *mental* stress prevention making you vulnerable to internalizing this stress into your stomach, adrenals, and immune system creating disease potential. You need nutrition for your nervous system, and affirmations to remain in mental balance and positive thinking. Your *emotional* stress prevention is moderate, and you may need reprogramming help. *[If needing help managing these stresses, see my prior books.]*

———

Love

Excess sulfur makes you crave affection: you need an understanding mate.

▶ *Rocine: "You need a non-demanding sexual partner, a devoted husband. You often mate with the carboferic, carbogenic, calciferic, isogenic, myogenic, and nitropheric types."*

———

Talents and Vocations

You are an avid learner and admire educated people. Your mind does not usually support long arduous studies.

Abilities - *Artistic, practical, managerial*

Found as character actors and occasionally stars, you are mostly artists, writers, designers, teachers, and in any refined, creative, or artistic work. Your type is ethical, honest, industrious, practical, hard working, and able to supervise others. The type information cannot predict what or who you will become, but you are capable of bringing a creative excellence or brilliance to whatever you do in life.

▶ *I have known or observed you as teachers, psychologists, dancers, actors—and one male transvestite who!*

Inabilities - *Scientific*

You have only a slight predisposition towards law, logic, science, medicine, philosophy, or mathematics. A therapist I knew lost interest in her profession; she was more into psychic healing.

———

Health Problems

When sick, your illnesses usually start with excessive cooked sulfur food intake. Your health problems or diseases usually occur in the following organs and tissues:

Skin — You may have acne and skin imperfections (from excess sulfur).

Throat — Is weak and liable to infection.

Sexual Organs — Diseases, cysts, tumors are quite common.

Spine and Joints — Are weak and easily injured; joint and spinal pains are customary.

Hypoglycemia — This is due to emotional and hormonal disorders involving the liver, pancreas, or adrenals.

Stomach and Intestines — A weak digestion tract is vulnerable to disorders, gas, constipation, etc.

Nervous Disorders — Conscious stress of everyday life internalizes in your organs producing immune system, adrenal, and gastro-intestinal problems.

———

Exesthesic Acid/Alkaline Factor

[See Chapter 3 for details on this subject, along with the common symptoms found with people of different nervous system dominance.]

For your health and healing, the genetics of your autonomic nervous system predispose you to needing a specific ratio of food acidity to alkalinity. You are born with an acid constitution requiring a predominantly **alkaline-ash** food intake for acid/alkaline balance. (Ash refers to the minerals left in your body after metabolizing foods.) Your autonomic nervous system dominance is *sympathetic.* Construct the following approximate ratio of food selections each day.

70% Fruits, salads, vegetables
30% Proteins, carbohydrates

▶ *Approximate your food ratios. On any particular day, it does not matter if one meal is mostly alkaline and another mostly acid—just try to balance it out for the day! If you make a mistake, try again tomorrow. It is a subjective call that you make. What is done over time makes the difference to your health.*

The Exesthesic Spiritual Factor

Skip this paragraph if uninterested in a philosophical perspective on your body type!

▶ *Rocine: "The soul chooses the body type."*

If as souls, we choose the brain and body type to spend a lifetime in, it could be to learn certain spiritual lessons related to perfecting ourselves, and our humanity, in God's eyes. What lessons does the type bring you? Only you can really decide what those lessons are. You know your weaknesses, faults, and behaviors towards others. You know things about yourself that Victor Rocine could never get from his research subjects when he first wrote about types. So search your mind for the answers.

Each discrete type has challenges of life lessons, spiritual goals, etc., and some of yours may be:

Temper — You need to become more calm and peaceful towards others, but how to do this. You are vulnerable to being somewhat emotionally explosive, which is in your DNA, in your wiring. A good therapist helps (along with stopping eating cooked sulfur foods).

Beauty, Sensuality — This is not really a problem unless you associate with people easily offended by your sensuous nature, or who are jealous of your beauty. Being beautiful and sensuous is in your DNA: it is who you are! You grew up around jealous women, and do not need to be around a jealous man! You need to work on differentiating between sexual and romantic love; your beauty attracts men so it is wise to make friends before making love! You need to answer the question as to why your soul chose to live in a shapely body over having a skinny, fat, or plain one. You need to separate your natural sensuality from love feelings.

Forgiveness — Forgiving may be a struggle; let God do the punishing.

Altitude — You like to control your life and the people around you!

If you relate to any of the above challenges, doing something to overcome them serves your evolution.

———

An Exesthesic Story…

I am always amazed how many body types are identifiable with a rear body view or by hearing a tone of voice or a laugh! Meryl's long legs, shapely figure and flowing dark hair, even from a rear view, identify her as an *exesthesic* type: elegant, exclusive, charming, intelligent, and sensual.

She complained of having a volcanic temperament and for no good reason blowing up at her husband and others. Her health base was fine and examination showed minor health problems, aches, and pains due to dietary problems. Her food intake showed excessive intake of cooked cauliflower, garlic, broccoli, turnips, spinach, mustard greens, and Brussels sprouts.

She stopped eating all cooked sulfur vegetables and ate *raw* sulfur foods, on alternate days, along with increased vegetable protein intake.

After two weeks on the above program, her husband came into the office to thank me for her emotional recovery! She continued to be fine as long as she followed the type eating requirements.

———

Exesthesic Type
Mineral Food Needs

Apply this mineral data to the diet following the Thin type descriptions.

Excessive Foods:
- *Sulfur (cooked)*
- *Calcium*

Deficient Foods:
- *Sulfur (raw)*
- *Phosphorus*
- *Magnesium*
- *Manganese*
- *Potassium*
- *Sodium*

These common deficiencies in your type predispose you to ill-health. If ill, be sure to use these lists with your daily food intake. If not ill, eat from the food lists 3-4 days weekly for health maintenance. All food lists are in descending order of concentration and value to you, choose servings of foods in the upper half of each list first! One serving is ½ cup.

Excessive Foods –

Sulfur in *cooked* form is excessive in your tissues resulting in sulfur acids, emotional instability, and bizarre symptoms. If you have illness or disease, eating raw sulfur foods (and avoiding cooked sulfur foods) is a significant healing factor.

Calcium is excessive in your tissues. It is highly concentrated in your bones, joints, muscles, nerves, heart, teeth, and gums; if you have an illness or disease calcium excess may be a significant problem.

―――――

Deficient Foods -

In illness or disease, it is important to correct these mineral deficiencies.

Sulfur from *raw* sulfur foods is deficient (see above note), and eating them helps your health and emotional balance.

Phosphorus is deficient and needed because of your intense nervous system activity and potential for brain exhaustion.

Magnesium is deficient and particularly important for your heart and digestive function.

Manganese is deficient and needed for strengthening weak tendons, joints, and muscles.

Potassium is deficient in your type. It is concentrated in and vital to the health of your muscles, heart, brain and all cells. If ill or diseased, potassium deficiency may be a significant healing factor.

Sodium is deficient in your type. Unsalted sodium foods are needed for all body types to help eliminate and prevent calcium deposition in joints, arteries, and soft tissues.

[See the Appendix for descriptions of mineral functions in the body.]

Note - The food recommendations are for the generic type. Additionally, you may need from a holistic healer or nutritionist something more specific for your individuality.

Minimize Excessive Foods

Sulfur (cooked): *0-1 times/week*

Cabbage, onions, cauliflower, garlic, Brussels sprouts, broccoli, turnips, mustard greens, rutabaga, spinach, carrots, eggs, shrimp, legumes, cauliflower, oatmeal, sorrel. [These acidic cooked foods are detrimental to your health. Avoid them and eat occasional raw sulfur foods only — 1-2 times/week.]

Calcium: *3-4 servings/week*

Kelp, cheese (Swiss, cottage, cheddar), turnip greens, carob flour, collard leaves, almonds, brewer's yeast, parsley, dandelion greens, Brazil nuts, watercress, dried figs, yogurt, beet greens, whole wheat, milk, seeds (sesame, sunflower).

Eat
Deficient Foods

Sulfur (raw): *only 1-2 servings/<u>week</u>*
Cabbage, onion, cauliflower, garlic, spinach, carrot, horseradish, radish, chestnut, coconut, orange, shrimp, asparagus

Phosphorus, Manganese:
1-2 servings/day
Seeds (pumpkin, squash), barley, rye, buck-- wheat, dry split peas, pinto beans, oats, goat cheese, peaches, cashews, beef liver, scallops, lentils, crab, lamb, mushrooms, whole grains, legumes, raisins, rhubarb, corn, alfalfa, endive.

Magnesium, Potassium, Sodium:
1-2 servings/day
Rice, cashews, filberts, scallops, lobster, cherries, blackberries, prunes, millet, buckwheat, rye, beets, kelp, celery, sprouts, strawberries, pine- apples, cranberries, avocados, yams.
[Note: Eat any other foods you desire, but be sure to include the type foods in your daily choices.]

Exesthesic Nutritional Supplements

- **Multi-Vitamins** — *[Take all supplements with food.] --2 capsules/ day*
- **Phosphorus** — *2 tablets/day ('Phosfood' from Standard Process Lab)*
- **Do <u>not</u> take extra Calcium** — *You already have excessive calcium in your body. (Exception: menopausal, osteoporosis, or on estrogen,)*
- **Magnesium** — *200 mg/ day*
- **Herbs** — *Brain detox – Chickweed or Gotu Kola Organ detox – Red Raspberry or Strawberry Leaf (Take one capsule, twice daily for one month; then one, three times weekly.)*
- **Evening Primrose/Flaxseed Oil** — *1 soft-gel/ day*
- **Other** — *Chlorophyll, blue-green algae, green magma, spirulina, alfalfa (Take daily as directed)*

Important Exesthesic Health Concerns

You need the v*egetarian* Food Guide following this description; any instinctive vegetarian cravings are normal for you.

▶ *Remember, you cannot live healthily on a flesh-based acid-ash (protein and carbohydrate) diet! Your diet should be about 70% alkaline-ash (fruits, salads, vegetables), or greater. You often choose to be vegan.*

Animal proteins should be limited to once weekly (or less). Your excessive flesh and cooked sulfur food intake makes you over-acid.

EXESTHESIC FACTORS

Aim for -
70% Fruits, salads, vegetables
30% Proteins, carbohydrates
and
50% Raw food diet
50% Cooked foods
Avoid cooked sulfur foods!
Take the recommended supplements.

Exesthesic Weight Loss

Losing weight depends upon you following the type instructions, summarized in this section.

- *Gluten* sensitivity is common
- *Stop* eating cooked sulfur foods (see list)
- *Protein* drink daily, about 25-30 grams
- *Eat* your body type deficient mineral foods daily
- *Follow* your *Exesthesic Guide (as above)*
- *Exercise*: your body type requires only light daily exercise (like yoga, walking, roller-skating, etc.)
- *Simple sugars*: stop all white table sugar and high-fructose corn syrup and drinks containing these sugars
- *Mental balance and positive thinking:* you are very easily mentally stressed by everyday life, which causes adrenal hypoglycemia, low blood sugar; you need to take these supplements: *calcium/magnesium*, two capsules, twice daily with food; and *chamomile,* two capsules with food
- *Hypoglycemia:* this hormonal imbalance stops fat loss, and usually initiates more fat production, so it is vital to deal with this problem: take *pantothenic acid,* 500

mg/twice daily with food (see my earlier books to resolve this problem)

- *Calories:* As with any dietary approach, calories in, must be *less than* calories out! Most markets sell a calorie booklet; make notes of your daily intake, and in most instances keep it under about 1500 calories/day

———

Thin Type
General Food Guide

(Vegetarian or Semi-Vegetarian)

Important Note

———

The Food Guide addresses the <u>Acid-Alkaline</u> aspect of your food intake, along with the <u>Type Mineral</u> factor presented throughout this book. It does <u>not</u> necessarily address calories or other dietary factors that may be pertinent to your personal health needs whether medical or appropriate for some other dietary need. So use your common sense and just include the factors described here with whatever healthy dietary choices you usually make.

For other nutrient information, consult with nutritional books or with holistic nutritional doctors. I particularly recommend the advice of Andrew Weil, M.D.

———

General Food Guide

This chapter presents a general Food Guide, upon which you superimpose the nutritional information from your type chapter.

———

Meat/Flesh Intake

Most muscle types should limit red meat to once or less weekly, while eggs, lamb, fish, or poultry are excellent in moderation. If ill or diseased, be sure to eat daily, one or two servings from each *deficient minerals* list. If not ill, eat them at least three times weekly for health maintenance. If this diet is similar to your present diet, but healing is sluggish, then:

- Decrease your carbohydrate and protein intake by about one-third
- Increase your fruit, salad, and vegetable intake by about one-third
- Consult with a holistic doctor, preferably one versed in nutritional and emotional evaluation

———

Over-Acid or Over-Alkaline?

Just as a log of wood burned in your fireplace leaves a mineral-ash, food ash refers to the minerals remaining after metabolizing foods in your tissues:

- Fruits, vegetables **alkalinize** tissues
- Proteins, carbohydrates **acidify** tissues

Usually You Are Over-Acid Due To:

- Excessive intake of dairy foods
- Excessive intake of proteins and carbohydrates
- Deficient intake of fruits, salads and vegetables
- Accumulated metabolic waste-acids (from years of eating excessive acid-ash foods, meats and carbohydrates, and from lack of exercise)
- You need to estimate the ratio of foods eaten. Generally, eat the following *approximate* ratios for your health:

> **70% <u>Alkaline-ash</u>** foods *(fruits, salads, vegetables)*
> **30% <u>Acid-ash</u>** foods *(complex carbohydrates like starches, grains, cereals, breads, flour products; and proteins)*

Approximate your food ratios. On any particular day, it does not matter if one meal is mostly alkaline, and another mostly acid—just try to balance it out for the day! If you get it wrong, try again tomorrow. It is a subjective call that you make, and it is what you do over weeks, months, or years that make the difference—not on any one or two days.

———

Important

- Minimize white sugar and alcohol intake.
- If desired, interchange lunches for dinners.
- Never eat foods you are allergic to, no matter what I recommend; if allergic, or suspect a food allergy, eliminate it and substitute from your type mineral lists.
- Eat the right foods 80-90% of the time and the Food Guide will work for you; unlike some types you do not have to live out of a health food store (although such foods are healthier for you).

▶ *Omit eating the excessive minerals in your type chapter, and be sure to eat one or two servings from the deficient list daily.*

Finally, in addition to your body type needs, other holistic healing matters also need your attention. I strongly suggest that you refer to my web site and earlier books for that information: *DrStenbeck.net*

———

Acid/Alkaline Genetics Chart

The following chart reflects each Muscle Type and its acid or alkaline-ash food needs. These ratios change if you are unhealthy or over age 45-50. On any particular day, it does not matter if one meal is mostly alkaline, and another mostly acid—just try to balance it out for the day! If you make a mistake, try again tomorrow. It is a subjective call that you make, and it is what you do over weeks, months, or years that make the difference—not on any one or two days or weeks.

———

Acid/Alkaline Genetics, Dietary-Ash, and Raw Food Needs

This chart shows the Rocine types, their acid or alkaline food needs, and the percentage of raw foods needed for your health and healing.

- Apply your Type Minerals to the Food Guide

Type Genetics	Acid/Alkaline Genetics	% Food-Ash Needed	% Raw Food
Atrophic	Acid	80% alkaline	90
Exesthesic	Acid	70% alkaline	70
Marasmic	Acid	60% alkaline	50
Neurogenic	Acid	70% alkaline	50
Pathoferic	Alkaline	50% alkaline	30
Sillevitic	Alkaline	50% alkaline	30

The above percentages vary depending on aging and the health of individual types.

▶ *Observe the excessive minerals in your type chapter, and be sure to eat one or two servings from the deficient list daily (or, several times weekly).*

———

Important

- Minimize white sugar and alcohol intake.
- If desired, interchange lunches for dinners.
- Never eat foods you are allergic to no matter what is recommended; if allergic or suspect a food allergy, eliminate it and substitute from your type mineral lists.
- Eat the right foods 80-90% of the time and the *Food Guide* will work for you.
- You may have allergies to wheat, corn, other grains, sugar, alcohol, and milk (examine your body reactions to these foods for fatigue, sinusitis, joint pain, skin rash, and gastro-intestinal reactions). Note that the *atrophic* type *requires* dairy foods for health and healing.
- Living out of a health food store is unnecessary (although such foods are healthier for you). If you want dietary perfection in your healing efforts, eat organic foods (from a health food store).

In addition to your body type needs other holistic healing matters also need your attention. I suggest that you refer to my web site and earlier books for that information: *DrStenbeck.net*

———

General Food Guide

[Superimpose the nutritional information from your Type Chapter into this Food Guide.]

Breakfast

FRUIT *salad, fresh (with citrus fruit) and* *protein: yogurt, kefir, milk, cheeses, or raw seeds or nuts* — *3+ times/week; or*

CEREALS *(whole grain), fruit, seeds, and nuts as desired* — *2+ times/week; or*

EGGS *(1-2) with lettuce, tomato, veges, non-wheat toast* — *0-3 times/week; or*

OTHER *choices* — *0-1 times/week*

Daily Liquids

Coffee, teas — *0-1 cups*
Pure water, citrus, fruit, or vegetable juices, soups, other — *as desired*
Wheat is a common allergy: avoid white breads; eat sour dough, millet, or oat breads instead.
Note: For in-between snacks, have fruit or vegetables, with seeds or nuts.

Food Guide
Lunch

SALADS, mixed green, with <u>protein</u> (cheese, soy, seeds, egg, etc.) Dressing: virgin olive oil and vinegar, low-fat dressings — 3-5 times weekly; and/ or

VEGETABLES with salad (and a <u>protein</u>: yogurt, cottage cheese...) — 1-3 times/ week; or

FRUIT salad (like breakfast)
— 1-2 times/ week; or

SANDWICH, whole grains, cheese and / or other non-flesh <u>protein</u>; small salad
— 0-2 times/ week; or

OTHER choices
— 0-1 times/ week

* Other oils less ideal; soybean oil is a common allergen; minimize commercial dressings.

Food Guide
Dinner

VEGETARIAN meals: include legumes, tofu, cheese, cottage cheese, seeds, nuts, egg, etc. (and/or salad) — 2+ times/week; or

POULTRY/FISH (3-6 oz.), salad and/or vegetables — 0-2 times/week; or

*WHOLE GRAIN PASTA, cooked (barley, rice, millet, etc.), and salad/or vegetables
— 0-2 times/week; or*

*OTHER choices
— 1-2 times weekly*

DESSERTS: Fruits, fresh or low-sugar desserts — as desired

Note: Be sure to include one or more selections from your type food lists in your daily food intake.

Note. Substitute flesh proteins with seeds, nuts, legumes, and other vegetables if *vegetarian.* You are vulnerable to being protein deficient so be careful to eat sufficient proteins and/or include a daily protein drink!

Food Guide Notes

Steamed Vegetables — Minerals are lost in the boiling of vegetables, so steaming or wok cooking is best.

Food Combinations — Eating proteins at the same meal with starches often results in indigestion, gas or constipation (as does eating fruit and starch together). For those of you with weak digestive systems, watch how this or other inharmonious combinations may be affecting you.

Periodic Detox Dieting — If you over-indulge in acid-ash foods, you need occasional elimination diets for tissue waste-acid removal, supervised by a nutritional doctor.

Minimize —
- Plums, cranberries, and their juices
- Commercial, sugared, and fatty salad dressings
- Red meats, processed meats, wines, alcohol, and milk
- Coffee, white sugar, fructose, and chemical sugar substitutes
- Exposure to drugs, environmental chemicals, pesticides
- Avoid eating allergic foods

Healthy Weight — You have a good ability to lose and control weight by following the Food Guide instructions. If you gain weight, the most common reason is liver or kidney irritation due to food allergies or negative emotions—the key is to eat non-allergic foods. The *atrophic and marasmic* types usually need to gain weight. (Obviously, if you have a medical condition that contradicts this advice, do not change your diet!)

———

In Conclusion

It is difficult to discern some *Thin* types from *Muscle* types (like the lean and strong *calciferic, nervimotive, and medeic* types). Study them well and you will see the differences.

———

Appendix

Brief Extracts from
<u>The 22 Unique Body Types</u>

Appendix A

Types
(Brief extract)

Type comes from 'typus' meaning an image or impression, the study of types being called typology.

▶ *Rocine: "A combination of mental and structural features is consistently found in people of the same type."*

Rocine wrote that all types are a mixture of positive and negative qualities. He based his work on the biochemical individuality of our *mineral* absorption and utilization. Of course, all minerals are absorbed, but he postulated that different types of people *selectively* absorb certain minerals, to a greater or lesser extent, requiring specific mineral foods for their enhanced health and healing.

▶ *The type information cannot predict what or who you will become, or how successful or not, but your type is capable of bringing a creative excellence to whatever you do in life. If your type has negative qualities that you disagree with, remember that they are only tendencies and may or may not manifest in you.*

This book enlarges on Rocine's premise (early 1900's), integrated with the later research of Herbert Sheldon, M.D., Ph.D., at Harvard University (1930's), along with my fifty years of observations and experience with this subject.

Comparing your shared physical (and sometimes psychological) descriptions with the Celebrity Lists further assists the identification of your type. It is not that you will look exactly like, or be a twin to, any particular celebrity. Look closely at a celebrity's features: face, profile, height, weight, head, etc. If you know something about their talents, beliefs, success and failure spheres, health and weight challenges, attitudes and behaviors, etc., then you get clues as to what your type may be.

––––––––

Understanding Types and Sub-Types

Each of us has a clearly discernible dominant type. Visualize the celebrity examples from movies, politics, sports, the arts and public life, and try to identify with their physical features. Look for similar features, remembering that you will not recognize all attributes in yourself. You are not looking for your twin!

The sub-type issue is the main reason people of the same major type can look so different. Remember that a type description does not characterize you exactly, but depicts your individual variant of a type.

———

Minerals

Minerals are essential life nutrients that accelerate enzyme and chemical reactions and provide a basis for your body typing. Although found in all tissues, different minerals tend to be concentrated in certain organs, their presence or absence contributing to the healing of such tissues; e.g., zinc accelerates prostate healing; calcium and manganese promote bone, joint and connective tissue healing.

Specific foods nurture each type, some people needing meats for their health others needing a vegetarian diet. A high potassium diet nurtures one person, while another needs high sulfur, calcium, zinc, or another mineral.

Mineral Digestion and Absorption

Compared to vitamins, minerals are *difficult* to digest, absorb, and utilize. In people with strong digestive systems, this aspect may not be important. The following factors should be in place for optimal mineral metabolism:

1. Stomach Hydrochloric Acid Production
2. Parathyroid Hormone Balance
3. Organ Toxic Metal and Chemical Removal
   [See details in <u>*The 22 Unique Body Types.*</u>*]*

———

Total Body Healing

Note that from a holistic healing perspective, in addition to minerals and type information, the following healing factors are necessary:

> *Nutrient Balance*
> *Mental Balance*
> *Emotional Balance*
> *Spiritual Balance*
> *Detoxifying Integrity*

The above factors are all important to your total healing especially if you are interested in self-healing (see my earlier books).

———

Appendix B

Researchers
(Brief extract)

The predominant workers in this area of human individuality from around 1880's to the 1960's are Herbert Sheldon, M.D., Ph.D., Roger Williams, Ph.D., and Victor Rocine, D.Sc.

Much information on Sheldon's research exists on-line and in medical psychology libraries; for interested readers there are other lines of research published in the last century. This present book is primarily about Rocine's body types.

Herbert Sheldon M.D., Ph.D.

In contrast to Rocine, Sheldon at Harvard University in the 1930's was trained in the scientific method and did painstaking research and publishing on human individuality. In comparing his findings with Rocine's work, a direct putative correlation is visible.

Roger J. Williams, Ph.D.

Another significant researcher in human individuality is the renowned scientist and biochemist, Roger J. Williams. He demonstrated that different people have varying levels of nutrients, enzymes, and other metabolic chemicals in their bloodstreams.

▶ *Williams's research firmly expands on the premise of individual nutritional needs in human beings. If interested in his research, I highly recommend his book <u>Biochemial Individuality</u>.*

Victor Rocine, D.Sc.

Note that when a negative feature is indicated, say neurotic tendencies, all members of the type are <u>not</u> that way; it is a type tendency reported by Rocine.

Rocine studied type-related diseases finding links between mineral and dietary factors with individual types and their diseases. In each body type, one or more dominant minerals are preferentially absorbed and utilized over other minerals.

He recognized discrete body types from their physical appearance finding genetically based mineral dominance to be the determining feature. He also correlated their physical features with psychological characteristics.

———

Appendix C

Genetics, Types, and Diet
(Brief extract)

This section deals with how nervous system genetics helps determine your eating choices for health: you are either born to be a predominant meat eater, a partial or complete vegetarian, or something between the two. The genetic factor determining this dietary aspect is the *sympathetic and parasympathetic* components of your central nervous system. This represents a basic factor in eating for health.

This chapter helps you understand your dietary inheritance, although instinctively, you may already have arrived there!

- If born **sympathetic** dominant you are *genetically acid*, desiring a predominantly *vegetarian* diet for your health (about 70% fruit, salad, vegetables to 30% proteins and carbohydrates).

- If born **parasympathetic** dominant you are *genetically alkaline*, desiring a predominantly *carnivorous* diet for your health (about 70% proteins, carbohydrates to 30% fruits, salads, vegetables). Few of you ever choose to become vegetarian because of the difficulty in satisfying your protein needs without meats.

- If born *intermediate* dominant you may eat food groups with little concern for the acid/alkaline factor. However, after age 40, you need a semi-vegetarian diet for healthy eating.

————

Chart of Relative Nervous System Dominance

In the following Chart, if you relate to many of the symptoms on one side you probably have that nervous system dominance; relating to both sides indicates *Intermediate* dominance.

If Vegetarian (Over-acid) --
Eat 70% fruits, salads, vegetables
And 30% proteins, carbohydrates

If Carnivore (Over-alkaline) --
Eat 70% proteins, carbohydrates
And 30% fruits, salads, vegetables

If Intermediate --
Eat 50:50 of acid and alkaline-ash foods

Make an *approximate* estimate of your daily acid and alkaline food intake (such ratios varying from type to type).

————

Symptoms of Relative Genetic Dominance

Vegetarians **(Over-acid)**	*Carnivores* **(Over-alkaline)**
Sympathetic Dominance	*Parasympathetic Dominance*
little or no flesh desire	*desire flesh*
easily constipated	*rarely constipated*
slow digestion	*fast digestion*
easily dehydrated	*not dehydrated*
strong thirst	*low thirst*
pale face	*flushed face*
high pulse after food	*slow pulse after food*
easy gag reflex	*slow gag reflex*
cool dry skin	*moist warm skin*
nervous stomach	*calm stomach*
little eyelid blinking	*much blinking*
nervous tendency	*mostly calm*
slower healing	*faster healing*
low oxygen-uptake	*good oxygen-uptake*
easily breathless	*seldom breathless*
insomnia common	*sleep easier*
few muscle cramps	*some night cramps*
calcium deposits rare	*get calcium deposits*

Appendix D

Help Identifying your Body Type with Dr. Stenbeck

If you desire help in identifying your body type, follow these instructions, and answer the questionnaire. For further information and fees, send me an email from page one of the website:

DrStenbeck.net

First name: _____

Country of birth: _____

Upload photos and send to the above website:

■ Head and shoulders: front and side views

■ Full body: front and side views

■ Also 1-2 teenage views

■ If possible, casual photos of mother, father, siblings

MY TYPE CLASS MAY BE: _____

(Thin, Muscle, or Fat)

AGE   -   _____

HEIGHT   -   _____ feet/inches

MY WEIGHT -   _____ pounds

Heaviest at age: _____

- Lightest as adult: _____

- Estimate age 15: _____

VISION - Excellent Average   Poor:

HAIR - Natural color: _____

    - Thin/thick? _____

    - balding? _____

SKIN - Quality: _____

    - History of acne, boils, other:

_____

_____

TEETH - Strong   Weak   Dentures

    - Cavity history: Many   Moderate Few

MUSCLES - Strong   Average   Weak

    Sports played _____

JOINTS   - Strong   Average   Weak

HEALTH - Childhood diseases?

_____

_____

- Adult diseases?

_____

AVERAGE DIET

- Beef _____ (times/week)

- Poultry _____ (times/week)

- Fish _____ (times/week)

- Eggs _____ (times/week)

- Water _____ (glasses/day):

- Vegetarian? Vegan? _____

- Other? _____

- Did your childhood diet differ? _____

The above will help me know who you are! I will send you a follow-up questionnaire for further help in identifying your body type.

Appendix E

On-line Health Consultation with Dr. Stenbeck

For further information, or to comment on this book, or to receive a response on any health issue from a holistic viewpoint, send an email inquiry from page one of my website:

DrStenbeck.net

Following that, I will suggest further healing needs, which we may pursue with an on-line consult.

———

Appendix F

Notes

See my book *The 22 Unique Body Types,* available at the usual online source, for further information and details on all of the 22 Types. The Appendix in that book has further information about:

Mineral Functions and Food Sources

Further Reading

———